Two free bonus books are included. Your books are presented in this order:

1) Mistresses Ultimate Collection of S&M and BDSM Rules for FEMALE Submissives and Slaves

2) The Absolutely Essential Guide to Erotic Breast Massage

3) Slave Sarah Is Getting 10 Hard Spankings Today: Volume 1(Mistress/female slave Dom/sub spanking story)

Mistresses Ultimate Collection of S&M and BDSM Rules for FEMALE Submissives and Slaves

---

This contract also comes in a 8.5" x 11" hardcopy size (entitled "<u>Mistress/slave BDSM Contract</u>") that has more room for amendments and additions. For your final contract you're probably going to want to get that.

Table of Contents

P. Play Rape
Q. Breast Bondage & Related
R. Punishments
S. Medical Play
T. Showering and Bathing
U. Massaging Mistress
V. Corner Time
W. Pulling Out Individual Pubic Hairs as Punishment
X. Unacceptable Behavior of the slave which includes Jealousy, Pouting, Being Bitchy,
Slovenly and Lazy
Y. Mistress Having Multiple Slaves
Z. Having Sex and playing with Others Besides Mistress
AA. Objectification
BB. Mummification (full plastic wrap)
CC. Blind Folds
DD. Pin Wheel Use
EE. Crossplaying
FF. Orgasm Denial
GG. Maid Service
HH. Gags
II. Strap-on Dildos & Vibrators
JJ. Mistress Being Taken with a Dildo/vibrator
KK. Handcuffs, Chains and Shackles
LL. Leather, Rubber or Latex Clothing
MM. Role Playing
NN. Cumming From Performing Cunnilingus on Mistress's Pussy
OO. Birth Control
PP. Tattoos, Branding, Piercing
QQ. None of the below activities are allowed without the consent of both parties, and on each occasion

Introduction

Reading this contract together can easily be your entertainment for one or more evenings.

By going through this contract you'll learn a lot about what BDSM experiences each person is into, or might be interested in getting into. Remember you can change the contract at anytime. There is extra space at the end of each section for you to write your own entries, if that is your wish.

Make sure to cross out and replace wording you don't want, then you both initial that entry.

This contract and its collection of rules are based on the Dominant being female and the submissive/slave being female.

The term *"slave"* in this book is used interchangeably with the terms *"sub"* and *"submissive"*.

The term *"Dominant"* is used interchangeably with *"Mistress"*.

Dominants may wish to test their submissive\slave on how well she remembers the rules and knows the specifics of the contract. (Good news, you now have a wonderful excuse to spank your slave if she forgets something from the contract!)

These rules are not presented in order of their importance.

Trust, care, mutual consent, safe sex practices, and general safety are absolute priorities. No matter what it's suggested that you incorporate at least the following into your playtime and lifestyle:

* Don't tie things around someone's neck, and no breath play, period!
* Create a "Safe word" for the submissive to say when (or if) things get too scary.

* Always be careful and take necessary safety precautions when engaging in BDSM activity. Keep proper medical facilities handy.
* Always insure that a bound person has adequate circulation. If the person tied up has to go to the bathroom or has physical problems, that person must be immediately released from bondage.
* Ask about medical issues before playing and adjust your playing activities according to any medical issues.
* Never leave anyone bound and alone.
* Understand what a gagged person sounds like in sexual ecstasy versus in pain.
* Do not play while under the influence of drugs or alcohol.
* Always check that your handcuffs and/or lock keys work before playing. If you have to go to the locksmith to get the handcuffs off, it's going to be embarrassing.
* When removing someone from bondage, allow them to move their own limbs.
* If pregnant or ill, check with your doctor before engaging in BDSM related activity.
*Always play within your own skill base and comfort level.

This collection is only a guide. You should add, subtract and adapt rules as desired. There is ample room for that. If you live with others, such as children, it's likely many rules will at least need to be adapted.

Mistress/slave BDSM Contract

(Feel free to change and adapt those areas of the contract as you see fit.)

I, _____ (slave), hereinafter referred to as "girl", agree to submit to

_____ hereinafter referred to as "Mistress".

The girl understands that her submission is voluntary and includes sexual submission, BDSM play including bondage and discipline subject to the terms and conditions set forth in this contract.

The girl and her Mistress agree to the terms as stated in this contract.

Having read and understood this contract, the Mistress and slave sign this contract freely and without reservation.

The term (length) of this contract is for _____ days from the date of signing.

MISTRESS	DATE
SLAVE	DATE
Witness (optional)	DATE

A. Rules Governing *Time In* and *Time Out* of this Contract

Definition of Time In: "Time In" refers to the period of time the girl is subject to terms and conditions of this contract. *Time In* is to be considered in effect at all times when the girl is in the Mistress's presence or communicating with her in any way.

Definition of Time Out: "Time Out" refers to specific periods of time when the girl is **not** subject to the terms and conditions of this contract. The following rules apply to this *"Time Out"* period:

1. Mistress may call a "Time Out" any time She wishes.

2. (This "Time out" can be for a specific period of time or an open-ended period of time.)

3. The girl may request a "Time Out" for a specific period of time only. The girl must state her reasons and the time period for the

request and await her Mistress's permission for the Time Out. Should her Mistress not grant the Time Out, her only option is to end her current relationship with her Mistress.

B. Mistress/slave Dynamics (Written from the perspective of the slave) *(Make changes by (1) crossing out the rule and writing into the contract its substitute in the blank space at the end of this section or (2) just crossing out the wording and writing in the new word or words above or below it. (Using white-out and writing over the white-out is an alternative also.)*

1. When Mistress speaks in person or online in chat, I will stop talking or typing immediately.

2. When in private, I will **always** call Her "Mistress", "Maam" or _____.

3. Unless not allowed to by my Mistress, in public I will put my hand around Her arm to show we are a couple. Mistress may instead want us to hold hands, do something else, or nothing at all.

4. I may not leave a conversation on the Internet or on the phone between myself and my Mistress without explaining what I need to do first and getting permission from my Mistress to leave. This is not the case if I'm cut off by the phone or Internet connection.

5. I, the slave will write down and keep on file any new rules Mistress adds to this list.

6. I will always answer immediately and sincerely every question that Mistress asks me.

7. I will always show my respect for my Mistress when in public. I want others to see how important my Mistress is to me.

When around vanilla strangers that I'll never see again it's ok to call Her (my Mistress) "Mistress" or "Maam", but around family or regular vanilla friends, I call Her by Her name. (In summary, I will address Mistress by Her name if I absolutely need to use a name; it's preferable that I use no name to address Mistress and only call Her "Mistress" or "Maam" but using Her name is okay if necessary.)

In the vanilla world, Mistress cannot require me to call Her (or someone else) in public by a title or name that would humiliate me. (I am the judge of what would humiliate me.) That can include calling Her "Mistress" in public.

8. Mistress's slave may not lie about her Mistress to others and vice versa.

9. I (the slave) am not allowed to lie to my Mistress or be dishonest with Her, ever. If Mistress asks me a question I will answer with complete honesty even though I think it could get me punished.

10. While with Mistress I will make a concerted effort to always look sexy for, and to act seductive with, my Mistress. My body after all is there for Her pleasure.

11. I will try to avoid looking at my Mistress's eyes straight on.

12. Sitting at the same level as my Mistress is to be avoided if possible. However in public this is difficult to.

13. Whenever I'm to be played with or otherwise taken, I will immediately take the position my Mistress orders me to be in.

14. It is my responsibility to clean off all sex toys with rubbing alcohol, soap and water after we use them.

15. I am never allowed to get out of any of my binds/shackles without permission when I'm being (or have been) tied up or shackled. The obvious exception is if there is an emergency, I am in undue pain and/or I am in some way in danger and/or in a position that puts me in danger.

16. Whenever I'm to be played with or otherwise taken, I will immediately take the position my Mistress orders (or has ordered) me to be in.

17. If I wish to say something to my Mistress that could be controversial or seem too forward, I will first ask for "permission to speak freely". If what I say is deemed by Mistress to be too controversial, or seem too forward, and I have not done this, I (the slave) accept that I could be punished.

18. Mistress always has the right to punish me if She thinks I deserve it.

C. What I (the slave, i.e. the girl) Will Wear *(Written from the perspective of the slave) (Make changes by (1) crossing out the rule and writing into the contract its substitute in the blank space at the end of this section or (2) just crossing out the wording and writing in the new word or words above or below it. (Using white-out and writing over the white-out is an alternative also.)*

1. Mistress has the final say on what I wear when I am with Her and that includes when we are in public and in private. In private with my Mistress I should feel uncomfortable when fully clothed. I am in essence hiding myself from Her. The exceptions to this would be if we're expecting company and/or if it's cold.

2. Mistress can decide what I'm going to wear even though we're not going to be together at that time period. What I wear however must not humiliate me or be a danger to me.

3. I am required to dress feminine and/or in role play oriented clothing at all times unless ordered not to. The exception would be if I need to dress differently for work or another public/vanilla activity of some sort.

4. Nothing loose! I will look sexy at all times. I will wear make-up. I know how important giving pleasure to my Mistress is and looking sexy gives Mistress pleasure.

5. I may *never* wear panties while in Mistress's dwelling (or our mutual home), except to take them off when entering, and in preparation to go out. Of course the exception is when I'm given permission to wear panties in the dwelling.

6. I wear dresses or skirts only unless granted permission otherwise.

7. I will make a concerted effort to procure role play outfits that my Mistress enjoys. If I have it, my schoolgirl outfit and other types of BDSM role play outfits should always be ready to wear when at my Mistress' dwelling.

8. When in private, (alone with Mistress,) if I want to put any clothing on, even a bra or panties, I will ask permission from my Mistress first.

D. Rights of the girl (the slave). *(Make changes by (1) crossing out the rule and writing into the contract its substitute in the blank space at the end of this section or (2) just crossing out the wording and writing in the new word or words above or below it. (Using white-out and writing over the white-out is an alternative also.)*

1. The girl (i.e. the slave) has the right to expect her Mistress to love, cherish and safeguard her well-being during the period of this contract.

2. The girl has the right to privacy. She will not be required to exhibit or provide her submissiveness and/or naked body to others unless she has given full and knowledgeable consent to her Mistress.

3. Only those who she (the slave) chooses to be made aware of this contract and/or any of its contents, will be made aware of it. This includes family, friends, business associates and neighbors.

4. The girl reserves the right to decide who may or may not be made aware of her interest in BDSM and her submission to her Mistress.

5. The girl has the right to expect her Mistress to be knowledgeable in the Dominant/submissive lifestyle and to ensure her safety and well-being while participating in any physical activity.

6. The girl has the right to refuse to participate in any activity, at anytime, which she feels will cause her harm, jeopardize her safety or cause her emotional stress.

7. The girl has the right to expect that the requirements of her Mistress will take into consideration her lifestyle and her business situation and adjust to them accordingly.

8. The girl has the right to ask for an adjustment or modification to the terms of this contract at any time. These adjustment(s) must be mutually agreed upon with her Mistress or the girl's only recourse is to agree to not require said adjustment(s) or modification(s) or instead to terminate the relationship with her Mistress.

9. The girl and/or her Mistress have the right to cancel this contract at any time with a simple notification to the other.

10. The girl has to right to expect her Mistress to know her, who she is and has always been, and to respect these facets of her personality and not to require her to do, or become anything which would make her uncomfortable or in any way interfere with those facets of her personality.

11. When around vanilla strangers that the girl likely never will see again, it's ok to call Her (my Mistress) "Mistress", but around family or regular vanilla friends, the girl calls Her by her name. (In summary, the girl will address Mistress by her name if she absolutely needs to use a name; it's preferable that she will use no name to address Mistress and only call her "maam" or "Mistress" but using her name is okay if necessary.)

In the vanilla world, Mistress cannot require the girl to call her, or someone else in public, by a title or name that would humiliate the girl. (The girl is the judge of what would humiliate her.) That can include calling Her "Mistress" in public.

12. The girl's Mistress may not steal from her and/or force her to commit an unlawful act.

13. Mistress may not steal from the girl and/or force the girl to commit an unlawful act.

14. Mistress's slave may not steal from her and/or force her to commit an unlawful act.

15. Mistress may not legally and/or illegally take advantage of Her slave financially.

16. Mistress's slave may not legally or illegally take advantage of Her Mistress financially.

17. Financial slavery is never allowed on any occasion.

E. How I (the Slave, i.e. the girl) Will Treat My Body
(Make changes by (1) crossing out the rule and writing into the contract its substitute in the blank space at the end of this section or (2) just crossing out the wording and writing in the new word or words above or below it. (Using white-out and writing over the white-out is an alternative also.)

1. I (the slave) will always treat my body well and protect it as it exists for my Mistress's pleasure and to harm it is not only bad for me but disrespectful of my Mistress. I will need permission from my Mistress to smoke cigarettes, do drugs, eat poorly, get too little sleep and/or other dangerous activities. For Instance, if I am cooking, I am required to wear an apron to protect my body, even if Mistress is not allowing me to wear clothing at that time. (Any Mistress that does not want her slave to protect her naked body around hot food is likely a bad Mistress and likely not a good Mistress to belong to!)

2. At anytime if Mistress feels I am no longer the most desirable weight, She can order me to actively lose weight. I will have to go on a diet and/or workout. She can be the TaskMistress concerning this and punish me if I am not trying to lose weight or trying hard enough. Exceptions will be if I am pregnant or overweight due to a medical condition.

F. Kissing *(Make changes by (1) crossing out the rule and writing into the contract its substitute in the blank space at the end of this section or (2) just crossing out the wording and writing in the new word or words above or below it. (Using white-out and writing over the white-out is an alternative also.)*

1. Mistress may kiss me on any part of my body anytime She wishes other than when it could embarrass or humiliate me. If I don't want Mistress to kiss me in front of my family, co-workers or boss, etc. then Mistress is not allowed to. In private Mistress may kiss any part of my body that She wishes and at anytime and as often as She wishes.

G. Rules Affecting Me Sexually As a Slave *(Make changes by (1) crossing out the rule and writing into the contract its substitute in the blank space at the end of this section or (2) just crossing out the wording and writing in the new word or words above or below it. (Using white-out and writing over the white-out is an alternative also.)*

1. In private, Mistress may remove (or have me remove) any or all of my clothing at anytime. As a slave, when in private with your Mistress, you should feel at least somewhat uncomfortable clothed as you are hiding yourself from your Mistress.

2. When I am in bed with my Mistress, and if She is awake, I will need permission from my Mistress to leave the bed.

3. When I and my Mistress are laying down for rest or sleep, I must lay in a way in the way that She instructs me too. This is likely to better make my body available for her pleasure.

4. My pussy should always be kept clean and fresh when with my Mistress. After all Mistress may wish to use it for her pleasure at anytime. If Mistress checks and my pussy is not smelling and/or tasting fresh and clean then I can expect to be punished.

5. I will exercise my pussy to keep it tight for Mistress's pleasure. I can be punished if my pussy is not tight enough.

While Mistress is playing with me (or at other times), She may order me to "tighten my pussy" for a reasonable period of time. Mistress should feel the difference in pussy tightness.

My pussy being tighter than most will be a source of pride for me and Mistress will reward me for having and keeping a tight pussy!

6. **When I'm being played with and at the same time Mistress orders me to cum, I will do so. I will cum longer or harder at Mistress's discretion. This called "Orgasm-on-demand" and may require some training.** When I orgasm, I orgasm for my Mistress. By orgasming I show Her that I respect Her and that I know I must obey Her. As Her slave, when I'm being played with, I have no choice but to orgasm often and as hard as my Mistress orders.

7. I may not touch my Mistress's pussy, ass or breasts ever without Her permission.

8. Unless told otherwise, while Mistress is sexually playing with me, I must always ask my Mistress for permission to cum unless I have already been given permission to start my orgasm.

Also, unless told otherwise, while Mistress is sexually playing with me, I must always ask my Mistress for permission to **STOP** cumming unless I have already been given permission to stop my orgasm.

9. While Mistress is taking me (meaning making me orgasm by some means), I will orgasm especially hard when Mistress is orgasming.

10. My body exists to please my Mistress - I must always be anxious and willing to cum for my Mistress.

11. I'm not required to do this regularly but should my Mistress order me to, I will thank Her for allowing me to cum after I have orgasmed.

12. When my Mistress's hand, hands or mouth moves toward my pussy I will always instinctively spread my legs.

13. When my Mistress's hand or hands moves toward my breasts I will instinctively move my arms and stick out my chest to make my breasts as available as possible as they belong to my Mistress and are there for Her pleasure.

14. When in private, if Mistress wants any of Her friends to spank me, while clothed or in my panties, I will comply and not resist during the spanking. I have the final say if this person will spank me on my bare bottom. If the spanking is too hard and/or that person is disrespectful, I have the right to end this experience at anytime.

15. It is my decision as the slave as to whether I will rim (eat out) Mistress' or anyone else's anus.

H. Cunningilus of the slave *(Make changes by (1) crossing out the rule and writing into the contract its substitute in the blank space at the end of this section or (2) just crossing out the wording and writing in the new word or words above or below it. (Using white-out and writing over the white-out is an alternative also.)*

1. Option 1: Mistress will not eat my pussy as part of sex. Mistress would only eats my pussy as a reward, or as a special occasion such as a celebration. Having my pussy eaten is something I earn. When Mistress eats my pussy I will orgasm especially hard from it.

2. Option 2: Mistress likes my pussy juice and Her slave will be required to provide Her with as much pussy juice as She demands. When in private, at anytime, Mistress may say "pussy juice" or something like "I want pussy juice" and Her slave will quickly remove her cloths from at least her waist down and take a position where it is easiest for her Mistress to lap down her pussy juice.

As long as they're in private, when a slave's pussy will be played with, including eaten, is the Mistress's decision not the slave's. Her job is to keep her pussy clean and fresh and available.

If the slave is so rude as to not provide her Mistress with an adequate amount of pussy juice, (and it is her Mistress not her that will determine if it's an adequate amount), then she will have earned herself punishment. The slave's body exists to give her Mistress pleasure so refusing to do such a thing is not allowed.

I. Cunnilingus and Pussy Worship *(Make changes by (1) crossing out the rule and writing into the contract its substitute in the blank space at the end of this section or (2) just crossing out the wording and writing in the new word or words above or below it. (Using white-out and writing over the white-out is an alternative also.)*

1. When alone with Mistress, unless She (my Mistress) has told me to do otherwise, I am to ask to eat Her pussy every 30 minutes or so if we're playing, every 60 minutes or so if we're not. How long I will eat Her is up to Her always.

2. NO teeth ever be felt on Mistress's pussy (unless She wants it) or I'll be punished, then I will resume eating my Mistress's pussy. This can be repeated an unlimited number of times.

3. If Mistress says "**head up**" while I am eating Her, I will stop eating Her and pull my mouth off of Her pussy and wait for her next command.

4. When told to keep my eyes down, I will look only at Her pussy, whether She is clothed or not, until told otherwise. Mistress will say "released" or something like it, then I may raise my eyes and go about my business.

5. When I am eating Mistress's pussy it is not my decision as to when to stop but my Mistress' decision.

6. When kneeling in front of Mistress, my eyes will be on her pussy, my legs at least somewhat spread and hands on Her thighs, rubbing Her thighs sensually and with great anticipation.

7. If we are in private and I am healthy, I will always obey my Mistress's order to eat her pussy.

8. The length of time I eat Her pussy is up to Her. Literally how I eat her pussy is up to her also. If any of my body parts are in pain from this activity, I will stop and tell Mistress about it. She will them allow me to rest. Should Mistress not allow me to rest, chances are he is a bad Mistress and I need to find another Mistress.

9. When spending the night, or more than a couple of hours in bed with my Mistress, I may not leave the bed before asking to eat Mistress's pussy first (unless Mistress gives me permission to otherwise leave the bed.)

10. Pussy Worship - If I determine I have the free time in life and if Mistress okays it, I will spend perhaps hours at a time, kissing, sucking, licking, eating, looking at, touching and loving Mistress' pussy and anus. I'm doing this for relaxation so I may think of other things about my life as I do it. Mistress's pleasure is not a priority during this.

Perhaps this is best considered a form of meditation. Mistress may be watching television, resting or reading. I will be in my own little world, worshiping Mistress's pussy.

J. The Collar *(Make changes by (1) crossing out the rule and writing into the contract its substitute in the blank space at the end of this section or (2) just crossing out the wording and writing in the new word or words above or below it. (Using white-out and writing over the white-out is an alternative also.)*

1. There is the private collar and the public collar. No one needs to know that the public collar is anything more than a necklace. My public collar could be a vanilla looking necklace but the private collar would clearly be a BDSM collar meant to aid in our playtime and my submission.

2. I will wear my public collar at all times other than perhaps when showering or when I need to temporarily wear something else for a special occasion.

3. When in private, Mistress decides when I should wear my private collar versus my public collar. If Mistress has not said anything regarding this, or has not previously made a rule about it, I will continue to wear my public collar in private.

K. Spankings *(Make changes by (1) crossing out the rule and writing into the contract its substitute in the blank space at the end of this section or (2) just crossing out the wording and writing in the new word or words above or below it. (Using white-out and writing over the white-out is an alternative also.)*

A normal, good quality spanking will leave a submissive's/slave's bottom a nice shade of pink or red. This is what a slave should expect, if not hope for. If necessary however, such a spanking should be worked up to.

1. Being spanked is a very important part of my relationship with Mistress, as well as therapeutic for me as a slave. I will beg Mistress to spank me often. I will have favorite implements to be spanked by so if Mistress allows me to pick an implement to be spanked by, I will be ready to bring it (them) to Her. When ordered to I (1) will beg to be spanked and (2) afterwards I will thank Mistress, (or whoever she is having spank me,) for taking the trouble of spanking me.

2. I will without hesitation take any position my Mistress orders me to should She wish to take me, spank me or otherwise play with me or punish me. I am never allowed to block my Mistress's spanks or try to get away from a position my Mistress has ordered me to be in unless there is an emergency or I am in harm's way. Should Mistress ever spank my hand because it was blocking a blow, I will be spanked much harder and longer (and/or be punished in other manners) and perhaps have my hands bound in front of me, if they are not already. I will also have the humiliation of knowing I was so disrespectful.

3. If Mistress orders me to hold any of my body parts still while She is spanking me, that is what I'm required to do.

4. Whenever I and/or Mistress and I come back from being in the public, I am to ask for a "returning from the public spanking." Mistress may order me to start and stop this at her will.

5. My pussy must be wet within 60 seconds into any spanking. No significant spanking will ever end at least until my pussy is wet.

6. If Mistress wishes She will train me to cum from being spanked. Most slaves can be trained to orgasm from being spanked and as a respectful slave I will learn to orgasm for my Mistress while being spanked. Within 120 seconds of the spanking starting, I will naturally start to orgasm (asking Mistress for permission to cum first of course). Also Mistress can instead order me to start my orgasm during the spanking at anytime 120 seconds or longer into the spanking. As always I will need permission to stop my orgasm, assuming I am still being spanked.

For training me to cum from being spanked, Mistress will likely start by using a vibrator on me during the spanking and ordering me to start orgasming just as he starts the vibrator that's on my clitoris.

Mistress acknowledges that I may need up to 10 training sessions with a vibrator in this manner. After then, should I disrespect my Mistress by not cumming while being spanked, (assuming I was given permission to cum,) then I will be punished.

7. During a spanking I may never try to block the blows or try to leave the position She has put me in. When I'm being bound or shackled I will not resist, however when I am being bound I may always tell my Mistress that it hurts in an unacceptable manner (if it hurts) so She can make any necessary changes.

8. Whenever I am to leave the house (apartment or where ever) for more than just quickly going to the car, or something quick of that nature, whether I'm also leaving with Mistress or not, I will ask my Mistress for a "going out in the public spanking." This is over and above any other spankings I may have recently received. Mistress may order me to start and stop this at her will.

9. When alone with Mistress, unless She has told me to do otherwise, I am to ask every hour, at the beginning of the hour, to be spanked for "my hourly spanking," no matter whether I've been spanked recently or not. Mistress may not want to spank me but I'm required to ask roughly on the start of each hour anyway. Mistress may order me to start and stop this at her will.

10. Any crying I do while being spanked (if I need to cry at all) will simply be a turn on for my Mistress and will not affect the length or to an extent, intensity of my punishment. If I cry while being punished it likely means I'm learning my lesson and am getting what I deserved. The exception is when I'm experiencing physical pain from other correctable sources. For instances if my hands are tied and my shoulder is in a painful position, I should always feel free to tell Mistress about that and Mistress is obligated to immediately take me out of the situation that caused

me that pain. Reasonable pain from being spanked however is not something that can be negotiated (assuming this point has been agreed upon by both parties.) If I do not like the kind of pain my Mistress ever gives me directly from being spanked, I need to find another Mistress or leave the BDSM lifestyle.

11. The duration and intensity of a spanking and what my Mistress uses on my bottom is always the choice of my Mistress. I may however discuss something that concerns me at anytime regarding this.

12. When Mistress and I are together, if I feel that I am getting into a bad mood, I'm to immediately ask for a "mood correction spanking" from my Mistress. This rule is repeated every five minutes until the mood changes. Should Mistress think I need yet another mood correction spanking and I fail to ask for another spanking within 5 minutes, I will receive a caning instead, and/or be put in the corner and/or be put in a cage and/or be tied/shackled alone somewhere else.

13. No blood or blisters from being spanked or otherwise beaten. If something of that nature occurs by accident it can be forgiven by the slave if she wishes. It also depends on how fragile the slave's body is.

14. I must give my okay for Mistress to spank me anywhere other than my buttocks. (See separate rules concerning flogging my breasts.) I acknowledge that sometimes my upper legs will get spanked as well as my buttocks and I give my okay to that.

L. Foreplay *(Make changes by (1) crossing out the rule and writing into the contract its substitute in the blank space at the end of this section or (2) just crossing out the wording and writing in the new word or words above or below it. (Using white-out and writing over the white-out is an alternative also.)*

1. As She prepares to take me or otherwise have me for Her pleasure, Mistress determines what our foreplay will be. I am allowed to make suggestions as to what to include in foreplay and always allowed to tell Mistress if something makes me uncomfortable or hurts.

Mistress might like me to kneel naked on the floor by the bed, chair or couch in preparation for me being taken or otherwise played with. I'll remove Her clothing when ordered to, climb on the bed and give Mistress a massage, including a butt massage. Again Mistress determines what part of Her I massage and how long I massage any part of Her.

Mistress may then turn over and I will turn my attention to Mistress's beautiful pussy when ordered to.

M. Miscellaneous Physical (including sexual) Orders I (the girl, i.e. the slave) Will Obey *(Make changes by (1) crossing out the rule and writing into the contract its substitute in the blank space at the end of this section or (2) just crossing out the wording and writing in the new word or words above or below it. (Using white-out and writing over the white-out is an alternative also.)*

1. When I am laying on my stomach for any reason and my Mistress says "elbows", I am to raise my upper body up on my elbows so my breasts are readily available to my Mistress to reach under my torso and play with. My elbows must not block access to my breasts. My breasts after all are my Mistress's property.

2. If I am kneeling or sitting on a hard surface, including a carpeted surface, Mistress will make sure I am on a lot of padding.

3. When I am crawling, perhaps while being lead naked by a leash, I will mainly be crawling on padded surfaces (such as carpeting) so as to not harm myself. Crawling on the floor for a short distance is okay.

4. While with Mistress, if my Mistress ever says "kneel in front of the bed", unless She points out a particular spot to kneel at, I am to automatically assume I am to immediately go to the pad on the floor next to the bed and kneel on it waiting for his further instructions. My eyes are to be looking down on the bed and staying that way until Mistress releases me.

If Mistress just says "kneel" I will kneel in front of Her wherever She is and wait for Her next instructions. My eyes will be on Her pussy (or Her clothed midsection) as I hope to be eating it soon.

N. Anal Sex *(Make changes by (1) crossing out the rule and writing into the contract its substitute in the blank space at the end of this section or (2) just crossing out the wording and writing in the new word or words above or below it. (Using white-out and writing over the white-out is an alternative also.)*

1. Once I have given my Mistress permission in our relationship to take me anally at anytime, She may at anytime take me or otherwise play with me anally (after I'm lubed up real well).

Has the slave given such permission now?

Yes_____ (if so the slave must initial it): _____ .

2. I have the right at anytime to require Mistress to put more lubrication in my anus and/or on Her finger, fist or toys she'll use in me, if I feel there is not enough lubrication. Mistress may never re-enter my pussy with something after entering my anus with that thing, prior to it being cleaned very well, as infections can occur that way.

3. As just noted, Mistress may insert toys into my anus as She plays with me but no toy touching my anus may be used for any other purpose until I have cleaned it thoroughly with rubbing alcohol, soap and water.

4. Mistress may insert a (finger for finger-fucking) into my anus if his finger nail is well manicured and clipped, lubricated and it will not harm my anus.

O. Pussy unshaved, unshaven and if unshaved, it's appearance *(Make changes by (1) crossing out the rule and writing into the contract its substitute in the blank space at the end of this section or (2) just crossing out the wording and writing in the new word or words above or below it. (Using white-out and writing over the white-out is an alternative also.)*

1. It is Mistress's decision on whether Her slave's pussy is shaved or unshaved, trimmed or untrimmed and if trimmed to what extent and what the design is. The slave has final say in regard to any waxing.

2. I will keep the area by my pussy clean and shaven as per my Mistress instructions.

P. Play Rape *(Make changes by (1) crossing out the rule and writing into the contract its substitute in the blank space at the end of this section or (2) just crossing out the wording and writing in the new word or words above or below it. (Using white-out and writing over the white-out is an alternative also.)*

1. I hereby give Mistress permission to include Play Rape at any point during our playtimes. I will not resist unless ordered to as that could give Mistress the wrong impression as to if I'm enjoying it or not it. I likely will also be bound as She takes me. I may be allowed to resist only from the waist up.

Q. Breast Bondage & Related *(Make changes by (1) crossing out the rule and writing into the contract its substitute in the blank space at the end of this section or (2) just crossing out the wording and writing in the new word or words above or below it. (Using white-out and writing over the white-out is an alternative also.)*

1. In private Mistress has access to my breasts at anytime. I will take whatever position Mistress orders me to so as to make my breasts more easily and readily accessible to Her.

2. When Mistress flogs my breasts I expect my nipples to become erect, my breasts to perhaps become some shade of red and tender if flogged for a lengthy period. I understand that flogging my breasts may become an integral part of our playtime. I have the final say as to what Mistress can spank my breasts with and how long my breasts are spanked.

No blood or blisters. Unless I bruise easily (which often also means the bruises go away quickly also,) bruising is to be avoided with any playtime activity.

3. Mistress may use my breasts for safe breast bondage.

4. If I allow it, Mistress may drip melted wax on my naked breasts as I am tied down (or in any position that She wants.)

R. Punishments *(Make changes by (1) crossing out the rule and writing into the contract its substitute in the blank space at the end of this section or (2) just crossing out the wording and writing in the new word or words above or below it. (Using white-out and writing over the white-out is an alternative also.)*

As previously noted, Mistress always has the right to punish me if She thinks I deserve it.

A list of ways Mistress can punish me can be added here.

S. Medical Play *(Make changes by (1) crossing out the rule and writing into the contract its substitute in the blank space at the end of this section or (2) just crossing out the wording and writing in the new word or words above or below it. (Using white-out and writing over the white-out is an alternative also.)*

Safe medical scenes/gyno play utilizing the slave as the patient is allowed whenever the Mistress wants it but the slave has the final say on what can be done to her.

T. Showering and Bathing *(Make changes by (1) crossing out the rule and writing into the contract its substitute in the blank space at the end of this section or (2) just crossing out the wording and writing in the new word or words above or below it. (Using white-out and writing over the white-out is an alternative also.)*

1. Mistress may order me to shower or take a bath at anytime that She wishes. I will smell fresh and clean from it or be punished.

2. Mistress may order me to shower or bath with her at anytime that She wishes. Mistress may bath me as She wishes, assuming it does not put me in danger.

3. I cannot be ordered by Mistress to bath naked with another person if I don't want to. Mistress may order me to bath him or her while I am clothed though. I don't need to touch their private parts if I don't want to.

4. If I am bathing or showering with Mistress, She has the right to require me to scrub him or otherwise bath Her and/or play with Her as to her specifications.

U. Massaging Mistress *(Make changes by (1) crossing out the rule and writing into the contract its substitute in the blank space at the end of this section or (2) just crossing out the wording and writing in the new word or words above or below it. (Using white-out and writing over the white-out is an alternative also.)*

1. If in private, at anytime, Mistress can order me to massage Her in wherever way She wishes. Mistress determines the length of the massage, its intensity, what body parts I massage and what I'll be wearing (or not wearing) while massaging. I might be giving Mistress long breast and butt massages!

V. Corner Time *(Make changes by (1) crossing out the rule and writing into the contract its substitute in the blank space at the end of this section or (2) just crossing out the wording and writing in* *the new word or words above or below it. (Using white-out and writing over the white-out is an alternative also.)*

1. When my Mistress requires me to do corner time, I will be positioned in the corner, naked, unless otherwise decided by my Mistress. I will go there immediately without resisting.

If possible my hands may be tied together to the ceiling above my head, and my legs may be tied to a leg spreader bar. I may or may not be spanked during corner time and I may or may not be required to cum (from the use of dildos, fingers or vibrators on me) for my Mistress during corner time. My Mistress will determine how long my corner time is and how often I am to be spanked while there and how often I will be required to cum, if at all.

If I need to go to the bathroom or have physical problems, Mistress is required to release me from corner time to satisfy those problems. I then can be returned to corner time if Mistress wishes.

W. Pulling Out Individual Pubic Hairs as Punishment
(Make changes by (1) crossing out the rule and writing into the contract its substitute in the blank space at the end of this section or (2) just crossing out the wording and writing in the new word or words above or below it. (Using white-out and writing over the white-out is an alternative also.)

1. As punishment, if I allow it, Mistress, using a tweezers and magnifying glass, can pull out individual pubic hairs. I may or may not be tied down for this punishment.

X. Unacceptable Behavior of the slave which includes Jealousy, Pouting, Being Bitchy, Slovenly and Lazy *(Make changes by (1) crossing out the rule and writing into the contract its substitute in the blank space at the end of this section or (2) just crossing out the wording and writing in the new word or words* *above or below it. (Using white-out and writing over the white-out is an alternative also.)*

1. Acting in the above manner will be a recipe for punishment.

Y. Mistress Having Multiple Slaves *(Make changes by (1) crossing out the rule and writing into the contract its substitute in the blank space at the end of this section or (2) just crossing out the wording and writing in the new word or words above or below it. (Using white-out and writing over the white-out is an alternative also.)*

1. If I agree to it, Mistress may have one or more additional female and male slaves, of which I am one.

2. Once I agree to it, when in private, Mistress can order me to play with her other slave(s) in the manner that She wishes. Mistress can also play/have sex with us all at the same time (and separately) if the proper sanitation and contraceptive precautions are being adhered to.

3. I will not be jealous of the attention the other slave(s) gets which includes Mistress' sexual favors. I will expect to be punished if I get jealous of Mistress giving Her other slave(s) attention.

4. If I am playing with the other slave I will take her/his pleasure and needs very seriously, as she/he is also required to do with me.

5. All of Mistress's slaves will need permission to play with each other. Sometimes I will be the dominant person when playing with the other slave and vice versa. That will be Mistress' decision.

6. If She requires it, Mistress might require that a slave ask Her permission before using a blindfold, gag and/or other play toys on another of her slaves during slave-slave play.

7. I will care about my Mistress' other slave(s) life as well as my Mistress'.

Z. Having Sex and playing with Others Besides Mistress

If I allow it, others at my Mistress's discretion may kiss me, touch and/or otherwise play with my sexual private parts as my Mistress sees fit. If I allow it, Mistress may order me to suck on somebody's cock, eat their pussy, have intercourse with them, make out with them, kiss them and/or bath them.

If I allow it, others at my Mistress's discretion may use me for purposes of BDSM play.

AA. Objectification (Objectification is requiring the slave to act like an object, such as a footstool.) *(Make changes by (1) crossing out the rule and writing into the contract its substitute in the blank space at the end of this section or (2) just crossing out the wording and writing in the new word or words above or below it. (Using white-out and writing over the white-out is an alternative also.)*

If both parties agree to it, provide more specifics here:

BB. Mummification (full plastic wrap) (This is the wrapping of the slave's body in plastic film [Saran Wrap type] from below the neck down to as far as the toes.) *(Make changes by (1) crossing out the rule and writing into the contract its substitute in the blank space at the end of this section or (2) just crossing out the wording and writing in the new word or words above or below it. (Using white-out and writing over the white-out is an alternative also.)*

Safe mummification of the slave from her shoulders down is allows at her Mistress's discretion.

CC. Blind Folds *(Make changes by (1) crossing out the rule and writing into the contract its substitute in the blank space at the end of this section or (2) just crossing out the wording and writing in the new word or words above or below it. (Using white-out and writing over the white-out is an alternative also.)*

The use of a blindfold on the slave by her Mistress can be done on any occasion if the slave allows it.

DD. Pin Wheel Use *(Make changes by (1) crossing out the rule and writing into the contract its substitute in the blank space at the end of this section or (2) just crossing out the wording and writing in the new word or words above or below it. (Using white-out and writing over the white-out is an alternative also.)*

Judicial use of the Wattenberg wheel (Pin Wheel) use on the slave's is allowed except for the following areas of her body:

a) anywhere in her pussy,

b) anyway from the neck up,

c) her knees

d)

e)

EE. Crossplaying (Crossplaying is where the slave is bound naked (or otherwise) to a large wooden cross and the Mistress does with her as She wishes.) *(Make changes by (1) crossing out the rule and writing into the contract its substitute in the blank space at the end of this section or (2) just crossing out the wording and writing in the new word or words above or below it. (Using white-out and writing over the white-out is an alternative also.)*

Safe crossplaying is allowed as Mistress desires it.

FF. Orgasm Denial *(Make changes by (1) crossing out the rule and writing into the contract its substitute in the blank space at the end of this section or (2) just crossing out the wording and writing in the new word or words above or below it. (Using white-out and writing over the white-out is an alternative also.)*

Orgasm Denial of Her slave is allowed to be done by her Mistress.

GG. Maid Service *(Make changes by (1) crossing out the rule and writing into the contract its substitute in the blank space at the end of this section or (2) just crossing out the wording and writing in the new word or words above or below it. (Using white-out and writing over the white-out is an alternative also.)*

Maid service will be provided at least semi-regularly by the slave if her Mistress wants it.

HH. Gags (Make changes by (1) crossing out the rule and writing into the contract its substitute in the blank space at the end of this section or (2) just crossing out the wording and writing in the new word or words above or below it. (Using white-out and writing over the white-out is an alternative also.)

Mistress may use a gag on Her slave. Her slave however has the right to not allow isolated instances of it.

II. Strap-on Dildos & Vibrators *(Make changes by (1) crossing out the rule and writing into the contract its substitute in the blank space at the end of this section or (2) just crossing out the wording and writing in the new word or words above or below it. (Using white-out and writing over the white-out is an alternative also.)*

Use of strap-on dildos and vibrators **are allowed** on the slave as well as when taking the slave in her pussy and ass.

When and how often these are used on the slave is the Mistress' decision.

If the strap-on touches or enters an anus, it may not be used on the slave in any way until it is thoroughly cleaned off as it is no longer sanitary anymore.

JJ. Mistress Being Taken with a Dildo/vibrator (Make changes by (1) crossing out the rule and writing into the contract its substitute in the blank space at the end of this section or (2) just crossing out the wording and writing in the new word or words above or below it. (Using white-out and writing over the white-out is an alternative also.)

If Mistress wishes it, Her slave(s) **will** use a strap-on or vibrator to play with and/or have intercourse in her Mistress.

KK. Handcuffs, Chains and Shackles *(Make changes by (1) crossing out the rule and writing into the contract its substitute in the blank space at the end of this section or (2) just crossing out the wording and writing in the new word or words above or below it. (Using white-out and writing over the white-out is an alternative also.)*

Handcuffing, chaining and shackling of the slave for purposes of bondage **is** allowed if done safely and in private. If not in private, the slave must okay it on each occurrence.

LL. Leather, Rubber or Latex Clothing *(Make changes by (1) crossing out the rule and writing into the contract its substitute in the blank space at the end of this section or (2) just crossing out the wording and writing in the new word or words above or below* *it. (Using white-out and writing over the white-out is an alternative also.)*

1. Mistress may require her slave to wear leather, rubber and/or latex clothing.

MM. Role Playing *(Make changes by (1) crossing out the rule and writing into the contract its substitute in the blank space at the end of this section or (2) just crossing out the wording and writing in the new word or words above or below it. (Using white-out and writing over the white-out is an alternative also.)*

Role playing (RP) is allowed. Allowable role playing scenarios are to be written in below. When the role playing will begin is always at the Mistress's discretion. (Any additional RP scenarios can be added at later times with both parties signing and dating the additions.)

1. When in private with her Mistress, and in a safe and private environment, and at her Mistress's discretion, the slave is required to wear any role play outfit Mistress wants her to (and that is available to them.) This includes school girl outfits, nursing uniform, etc.

2. Mistress will always have the final word as to how the role play outfit is worn.

Role Play Scenarios

A)

B)

C)

D)

E)

NN. Cumming From Performing Cunnilingus on Mistress *(Make changes by (1) crossing out the rule and writing into the contract its substitute in the blank space at the end of this section or (2) just crossing out the wording and writing in the new word or words above or below it. (Using white-out and writing over the white-out is an alternative also.)*

1. If Mistress requires it, Her slave will train herself to orgasm from just performing cunnilingus on her Mistress. Mistress must give her an adequate training period, including using a vibrator on her while she is performing cunnilingus but at some point if the slave is not cumming from giving her Mistress cunnilingus alone, she should expect to be punished.

OO. Birth Control *(Make changes by (1) crossing out the rule and writing into the contract its substitute in the blank space at the end of this section or (2) just crossing out the wording and writing in the new word or words above or below it. (Using white-out and writing over the white-out is an alternative also.)*

1. The slave promises to actively and aggressively guard her body from unwanted pregnancy.

PP. Tattoos, Branding, Piercing *(Make changes by (1) crossing out the rule and writing into the contract its substitute in the blank space at the end of this section or (2) just crossing out the wording and writing in the new word or words above or below it. (Using white-out and writing over the white-out is an alternative also.)*

1. I the slave will always have the final decision on whether I am going to have on my body any tattoos, branding, piercing or any other type of semi-permanent or permanent physical alterations. However, if I want to do any of the previously mentioned, but my Mistress doesn't want me to do it, then I am not allowed to do it.

Thus if I want to have a piercing but my Mistress won't allow it, I will not be able to get that piercing.

QQ. None of the below activities are allowed without the consent (on each occasion) of both parties:

Blood play
Knife play
Breath control (breathplay, asphyxiation)
Scat play
Urine play
Hypnosis of the slave
Forced cross-dressing
Forced homosexuality or bi-sexuality of the slave
Nipple torture
Spitting on the slave
Toilet play
Diaper play; Mistress's slave may not be required to wear a diaper.
Needle play
Electric Play (*Tens, Violet Wand and Shock devices*)
CBT (cock and ball torture)
Boot worship by the slave of her Mistress's boots
Kissing of clean boots/shoes of others
Verbal abuse
Ashtray play (When the slave makes herself like a table so her Mistress can put an ashtray on her back.)
Forced chastity
Sensory deprivation
Suspension/suspension play
Humiliation
Daddy/daughter
Forced 24/7 servitude of the slave.
Public exhibition of a slave
Pain enhancement of the slave
Ponygirl play (where the slaves pretends to be a pony, is dressed up as such and ridden.)
Duct tape use on the slave
Purposely stretching of any part of the slave's body

Forced confinement of the slave

Total Power Exchange (TPE) - (TPE is loosely defined as one person [the Mistress] completely, utterly and totally making the decisions for himself and his slave.)

Unusual mind control games

Rimming (licking, eating, and/or otherwise using the mouth/tongue on/in her Mistress's anus).

Fisting of the slave's pussy

Fisting of the slave's anus

Bestiality (This is illegal and bizarre. Don't do it.)

List Additional Rules Here:

The Absolutely Essential Guide to Erotic Breast Massage

Michelle Tallia

Extreme Pleasure Breast Massage

The specialized breast massage discussed in this book can give a woman more pleasure than she can imagine. If her lover is unavailable to pleasure her this way, women can easily give themselves *Extreme Pleasure Breast Massage*, and the great news is it's something women can do to themselves for the rest of their lives.

There are a great many positions a woman's body can be in to receive this specialized and very sexually arousing breast massage. For this example though, let's have her sitting up and at least topless. Do note however that as she gets more and more aroused, she'd probably prefer to be naked so one or both of you can access her pubic area with fingers or toys while she's getting Extreme Pleasure Breast Massage.

For this position the massager sits behind her and up against her back. If it's okay with who is getting the massage, I suggest the massager be naked as many women will lose control at some point when getting Extreme Pleasure Breast Massage and be anxiously reaching behind their lower backs to play with the massager's privates. If a woman has never experienced this type of erotic massage before, she in particular may react with callous abandon.

Before placing yourselves in any of the massage positions, you'll need to have readily available a good supply of quality lotion and/or massage oil. If using lotion, try to use some brand of non-desensitizing lotion. (Most lotions put desensitizers in them to dull the pain of dry skin and other irritations. These desensitizers can at least partially desensitize breasts thus cutting down on the breast's capacity to provide pleasure. Baby lotions at dollar stores sometimes are good ones to try but lotions tend to vary by brand. Another possibility to try is hair conditioner.) Cold lotion or massage oil on breasts can provide an unwelcome jolt so if warming is necessary, warm the lotion/oil up ahead of time. You can also rub blobs of it in your hands to warm it up. Always have an ample amount of this massage oil or lotion nearby as well as well as small towels to wipe the oil/lotion off of your hands and her breasts after the massage is over.

Put a sizeable glob of massage oil/lotion on each of your hands, rubbing it all over your hands to spread it out, as well as warm it if it's not yet warm. Then put your well lubricated hands on her breasts, *but not yet on her nipples and areolas*. This is because those provide the most pleasure and thus the best is saved for last!

It is so important that the massager make sure to keep his/her massaging hands *very* well lubricated. When the oil or lotion is breaking down the massager will feel stickiness developing. The rule of thumb is that you can't lubricate your hands and her breasts too much!

Also the massager needs to make sure his/her nails and skin of their hands are smooth. Trim and file your fingernails and that kind of thing, to as short and smooth as possible. Otherwise she (the person receiving the massage) might feel them as they rub against her sensitive skin. She can even get hurt by them because as she is in the thongs of ecstasy, she might not realize that they are hurting her, so make sure to watch out for her and take care of this situation.

Typically the massage will provide three levels of pleasure. (a) Massaging the fleshy part of her breast (but not massaging her areolas and nipples) should give her pronounced and very welcome pleasure; (of course the faster her breasts are massaged the more pleasure she'll get.) (b) Including her areolas in the massaging will increase her pleasure a lot. (c) But massaging her nipples and areolas at the same time will really get her going.

Below (and not in order of importance) are suggestions to optimize the breast massage.

* Start from the bottom of her breasts (where the breasts meet her torso) and work your way slowly higher up to just below her areolas. You can move your hands at varying speeds but typically the faster you massage the more pleasure she'll get.

* Simultaneously circle her boobs with each hand. Start out by using limited pressure on the breasts while utilizing only one finger, then gradually work your way up to utilizing all your fingers. Go clockwise then counterclockwise (or vice-versa.) Remember, *leave her nipples and areolas alone as much as possible until she's practically (or literally) begging for you to massage them.* Sure you will "bump" into them from time to time as you massage around them. Those bumps will give her a delicious taste of what's to come.

* At its base, wrap each hand around a single breast then run your well lubricated hands around and along that breast in a steady spiraling motion up the breasts in the direction of her nipples, until you reach the edge of her areolas. Of course you can go in the opposite direction also (starting from just below her areolas and working your way down to where her boobs meets her torso.)

* Place one hand on the base of one breast; the back of the hand should be facing her head. Put your other hand on the base of her *other* breast, the back of it should be facing her legs. Slide your well lubricated hands from left to right and then vice-versa, across and along both breasts.

* At its base, take each breast in a well lubricated hand and with increasing speed pull up from the base of her breast to the nipple until your fingers reach the edge of the areolas (or if you're already playing with her areolas and/or nipples, go all the way to her nipples.) Then do the opposite and slide your hands back down from the top of her breasts to the breast's base (where you started from.) Repeat this procedure many, many times.

* Tease her by sliding only your well lubricated fingertips over her breasts, wiggling your fingers.

* Instead of the above, perhaps for a minute or more, you'd like to start the festivities by teasing her breasts by only briefly touching them here and there using only the tips of your fingers.

* Concentrate your efforts on only one well lubricated breast; wrap both hands around it, kneading it, pulling it and twisting it.

As previously discussed, it's strongly suggested that you take your time before playing with her areolas and then nipples. This is because she will still get a good deal of pleasure from having the 'areola and nipple-less' massage. I for one require that she even beg you to play with her nipples--because as we know this is where the breasts offer the most pleasure. I would suggest waiting until she is already well stimulated. You may stroke her anticipation by whispering in her ear that you're about to play with her nipples, then suddenly do it. She may scream with delight as an orgasm overcomes her.

Playing with her nipples is typically the high point of her massage. She'll likely be getting the most pleasure now. (Again, the faster your well-lubricated fingers move around her nipples, the more pleasure she's likely to get.)

Okay massagers you now have a choice, you can immediately start massaging her nipples fast and hard, driving her crazy, or start massaging them slowly, then progressively massaging them faster and faster until she screams in ecstasy. If you're going to massage them fast immediately, as is the first option, many women will start their orgasm then (if they haven't already.)

Don't forget you can let her use a vibrator on herself as you massage her and thus it's suggested you keep a vibrator within arm's reach. Believe me she'll find it if it's there.

Because so often the woman you're massaging will get so aroused from all this that with both hands she'll instinctively reach around her lower back to play with the massager's pubic area. She then will not have a free hand to use the vibrator on herself. Of course both your hands are busy giving her Extreme Pleasure Breast Massage. A way to counter this is to secure a vibrator with white medical tape (the type used to hold gauge and cotton to cuts etc.) over her most sexually sensitive pubic area. (Perhaps it would be helpful if she keeps her panties on for extra support.) If you do this, more women will orgasm while you are giving her this massage.

Remember guys her nipples can get tender after orgasm and need to be left alone for a bit of time. Also don't over massage her nipples or they can get raw.

As is obvious, ladies, you can give yourself Extreme Pleasure Breast Massage in the privacy of your bedroom.

After the massage, ladies your breasts tend to become firmer for a while and often they'll feel quite good for hours.

The following is another way of giving this massage, (told from the perspective of the kinky dominant massager.) Warning it is kinky!

We will go to the bed (if we're not already there.) I will set the bed up so I am sitting with my back against the headboard of the bed and you are laying in front of me face-down on cushions with your head positioned so you can easily suck on my penis and play with my scrotum using your tied-together hands.

Also I'll put a roughly 3' x 3' sheet of plastic under your upper body to keep the massage lotion or oil from going on the bed covers. (More on this massage very soon!)

Perhaps I will also tie your bound hands to the headboard. If I do that though I will make sure there is enough slack in the rope for your hands to still move freely around my penis and scrotum while you suck. If your hands are tied to the headboard, I will be sitting on the rope as my butt will be in-between your bound hands and the headboard which your hands are tied to.

Your breasts will now be positioned, thanks to these cushions, just above the ground. As you suck on my penis, I will generously lubricate (and keep lubricated,) your breasts with some brand of preferably non-desensitizing lotion. I will warm the lotion/oil up ahead of time or rub it in my hands to warm it up, if warming is necessary. I will then massage your breasts. (Many lotions put desensitizers in them to dull the pain of dry skin. These can at least partially desensitize breasts thus cutting down on the breast's capacity to provide pleasure.) I will continue for a long time to massage your lubricated breasts as you suck on my penis. (This is known as "Extreme Pleasure Breast Massage". Remember to always keep the massager's hands well lubricated!)

Using a yardstick type implement, I can reach across your back and spank you as you suck. Obviously one should make sure the woman can handle being spanked while sucking. Most can depending on the intensity of the spanking and how hard she's already orgasming.

End

This book is sold and/or distributed with the understanding that the publisher and author is not engaged in rendering legal or other professional services. **This book and its subject matter is for entertainment purposes only.** In this publication there may be inadvertent inaccuracies including technical inaccuracies, typographical inaccuracies and other possible inaccuracies. **The writer and publisher of this publication expressly disclaim all liability for the use or interpretation by anybody of information contained in this publication.** The author, publisher and distributors of this publication hereby disclaim any and all liability for any loss or damage caused by errors or omissions resulted from negligence, accident, or any other causes. If legal advice or other expert assistance is required, the services of a competent professional person in a consultation capacity should be sought. Products, services and websites' content vary with time. Please verify any published information.

Slave Sarah Is Getting 10 Hard Spankings Today
Volume 1

By J. R.

Copyright (C) 2013

Hello I'm slave sarah. My mistress is very demanding and strict. She controls my life in almost every way. I pleasure my mistress many times a week. I'm also available to any of her friends if she wishes.

Depending on her mood and who is with us, I serve her in different ways. Mistress is a firm believer of keeping her slave well disciplined and has a big collection of paddles, slappers, straps, whips, floggers, heavy rulers and more. It's my job to keep them organized and in order. I also have to keep all her toys clean and organized.

Mistress spanks me on average about twice a day. It's something she genuinely loves to do. Usually mistress always gives me a spanking before bedtime. That spanking is among my favorite as it helps make me sleepy. If a friend comes over that's into BDSM she'll let him or her spank me also if they want. I don't think she thinks I can be spanked enough. I am not allowed to wear any cloths at home unless we are expecting vanilla company or if it's cold. I stay in my room usually anyway unless called. It's a nice room with a TV, computer and Internet. Mistress also has a cage in the basement that I get put in, often in preparation for playtime or if she's angry with me. When Mistress is horny I have to particularly be careful as she'll punish me for the smallest of things.

Mistress' friend Mistress Lynne came over for a visit yesterday and as usual I was tied up on the half table, spanked and taken with her strap-on. The half table is several feet long with stirrups so my legs are kept securely straight up in the air. My arms and lower pelvis are strapped down to the table. My d-cup breasts thus are securely in place should they be the focus of attention, as they often are. On the half table my pussy and asshole are right on the edge of the table so they can be taken with ease. When I'm being spanked on my tits or ass I usually will be required to cum at some point, which is no problem for me. While using the strap-on in my pussy Mistress Lynne finally let me cum and wow was that ever a great orgasm.

Typically in the morning I wake up and fix Mistress breakfast. She may call me into the bedroom to pleasure her if she is in the mood, particularly if it's the weekend. I may need to help her dress but usually while she is in her underwear or slip, she'll gives me a good over the knee spanking before she goes to work. She says it helps get her blood pumping and be more ready for the day. Those morning spankings can really wake me up fast. It's usually always with a paddle or strap. Mistress doesn't usually spank me with her open hand anymore, she used to several years ago. As Mistress is paddling me in the morning, she will tell me what she wants me to do that day, assuming there is something she has on her mind.

I have to admit that today was a different as Mistress started the day very angry with me. I was supposed to get more of her shampoo and lip stick when I went shopping yesterday but forgot. She found out as she was taking a shower. As she was drying off she called me in, ordered me to crawl from the bedroom door to the foot of the bed and was lecturing me about being forgetful. She hates it when I'm forgetful, frankly it's something I have a problem with. I knew I was in a lot of trouble. I could see she was winding up to really spank me hard. I apologized of course but that rarely does any good. She ordered me to set the chair up in the middle of the bedroom and get the large black wooden paddle. She ordered me to bend over the back of the chair so my hands were on the chair seat and my butt was the highest thing on me. I looked back at her as she came over, careful not to look at her eyes of course. What I saw made me cringe. She looked really mad. She was scolding me as she ordered me to count out the swats. She started by tapping my butt with the big paddle then, to my surprise put the large wooden paddle on the bed nearby and went and got the black leather strap. It was the first spanking implement we ever ordered together. It's falling apart a bit but still packs quite a punch. She started right in on my butt with it. Slap...slap...slap...SMACK, SMACK, BAM, BAM, SMACK, SMACK... Sure I'm required to hold still but it's not easy when she gets in a mood like this. I began moaning after the 7th spank or so then gave progressively louder yelps after the 15th. Usually though I can usually take a very hard spanking. Maybe my butts toughen up a bunch over the years.

Mistress kept scolding me about forgetfulness. She's had trouble with me about this before. Smack, smack..smack, BAM, BAM, BAM. My butt cheeks were bouncing around from the blows and getting redder and redder. Since Mistress was pressed for time I think she spanked faster and harder. After the 60th or so spank I was begging her to stop. "Ow mistress, pleaseee I'mmm soorrry." I was flinching and moving my outstretched butt something that unfortunately which made her madder. She grabbed me and held me in place as she really laid it on my ass. I knew it was getting red by then. SMACK, SMACK, BAM, BAM, SMACK, SMACK. Finally she stopped but instead went to get the big black wooden paddle, the one she had ordered me to bring in the first place. "Move away or block even a single blow and you'll spend the next two days in the cage slave." "Yes Maam". I meekly said holding on to the seat with all my might. BAM, BAM, BAM, BAM. "ow, ah, pleasseee, no moore mistress." BAM, BAM, SMACK, SMACK, BAM, slap…slap, slap. "What is my favorite color for your ass young lady?" Mistress howled. ""red maam," I sheepishly muttered as I softly cried. "I'm now going to check your pussy and god help you if you're not soaking wet". Mistress' rule was that I had no more than 30 seconds into a spanking to have a wet pussy. This spanking had lasted a lot longer than that already. She must have not woken up completely because she's usually checking me sooner than that. Mistress is always looking for a reason to punish me and that would be one of them. I felt her fingers enter my pussy and feel their way around inside of me, she teased my clit and I started to cum immediately but I'm a well trained slave and know better than to cum without permission. "Mistress, please may I cum, please, please." Of course she wouldn't let me cum then and her fingers withdrew, soaking wet. Mistress rubbed my hot red ass for a bit but I knew the only thing that would stop this spanking would be her not wanting to be late for work. That's one of the great things about our morning spankings. Mistress doesn't have a lot of time to complete them. "Stand up young lady" she ordered and I pushed myself up from the chair rubbing my sore butt. Mistress caught me rubbing myself. "Hands behind your back slave." Mistress then took the heavy wooden ruler in hand and sat on the chair I was just bent over. "Lay over my lap now." I quickly complied, my open palms on the carpet and my toes were also on the carpet. I would have to stay this way or the spanking would never stop. That was the rule. Mistress rubbed the heavy wooden ruler over my ass. "I love how red your ass gets from a good spanking" she said. "Thank you maam." I mumbled. The truth was that by rubbing the ruler over my well spanked ass like that, I was about to cum, but that sensation would abruptly change. BAM!! Wow no warm up but hard spanks right from the gitgo. BAM, BAM...SMACK, SMACK, BAM, slap...slap, smoosh, slap, bam, BAM. I was crying now. "No please Mistress, I'll be good, I swear." BAM, SMACK, SMACK, BAM, slap. Tears were willowing up in my eyes . ""Ow Maam, I'm sorry, I won't dooo it again, I swearr." Now mistress was spanking me in rapid succession. She really like spanking that way. The side and the top of the right cheek was getting most of the attention for 2 or 3 minutes then it was the left cheek's turn. After 40 or so really hard swats on each cheek, her spanking tempo slowed and her spanking intensity slowed. The end of this spanking was near. "There" Mistress finally stopped the deluge and looked down at her slave's reddening ass proudly. "A job well done. Get up. You may rub yourself." I stood up and furiously rubbed my butt. This was definitely a harder spanking for a morning spanking than usual; little did I know how much more was to come.

Mistress was already in her panties and ordered me to put her bra on. She then put on her dress then sent me to stand in the corner. I still was rubbing my ass but the sniffling had stopped. Mistress liked to hear me cry in some manner after receiving a good spanking. She came over to me on her way out of the bedroom. She pulled my hands away from my butt and started rubbing my hot red buttcheeks herself. Suddenly it dawned on me what could happen, I couldn't believe I had just thought of it. "I'm going to ask some folks to come over while I'm gone and have them also punish you. You will serve them also if they want. You will remain naked until I tell you differently." "Yes Mistress" I gulped.

Mistress knew many people in the BDSM scene. Several times before Mistress has had them come over to the house to punish me. I have also had to go to their places, typically in a short skirt and no panties, and get punished at their convenience. Sometimes we have bdsm parties and slaves like me would entertain the masters and mistresses. Those that allowed it would let their slaves be played with by the other dominants and submissives. Typically all the participating slaves would go one at a time to each master and mistress in the room and ask how they can serve them. Usually we would be spanked and have our pussies and tits played with. Some would require that we cum from it. We also would give hand jobs and blowjobs and eat pussy if they wanted it, and of course it would be our responsibility to clean up after the men came. There were vibrators and dildos all around and they would be used on us slaves by others as we kneeled in front of our betters. The lucky masters and mistresses though got to do a lot more with us later. I wanted to note that all going to these parties were required to be tested first for STDs.

After a female slave had gone around the room serving the Doms and FemDoms, she would be tied down on her back to a padded table, her pussy and anus on its edge, and the masters and mistresses would take turns taking her. All men were required to use condoms. I remember one night, while tied down, helpless and vulnerable, my pussy was taken 15 times. 6 masters took me once each, 3 masters took me twice and 3 mistresses used a strap-ons on me. That night my Mistress was not allowing anyone to take me in my ass, but some nights she would. My pussy would feel so hot afterwards. I suspect it was all the friction. Sometimes I would be sore for several days from this. Of course I had to cum for all of them which wasn't as easy later in the night but I didn't want to be punished. I should note that the masters weren't only taking me but also taking the other female slaves so they wouldn't spend as much time in me as they would normally.

Anyway, as Mistress was leaving she said that she would be back for lunch to punish me again and she would also send Master Terry over in the morning to punish me as well. Clearly this was going to be a long day. Happily Mistress released me from the corner as she walked out the front door and I now had some time to collect my thoughts.

Chapter Two

My butt heals fast, probably because it's been spanked so much. Its redness goes away surprisingly fast and frankly Mistress doesn't like that. She'd prefer watching me walk around the house naked with a well spanked, red, marked butt. Bruises show up on my butt but they too go away surprisingly fast. The fact is I would need all those physical characteristics to get through this incredibly spank-filled day.

I put the paddles, straps and other spanking implements away in the closet where they hang or lay in draws. I made Mistress' bed and tidied up her room. Mistress had ordered me to be naked so I didn't have to decide what to wear. I went to the kitchen and proceeded to clean it up. The biggest problem for me was that I was now horny and there was no way I could cum without a Dom or Domme's permission.

I laid down on my bed recalling the already busy morning when the phone ran. I saw it was mistress' number and quickly answered it. "I am going to take care of your forgetfulness once and for all young lady." Oh oh, this didn't sound good. "Today you will get spanked 10 times. And I mean good spankings, not love taps. If that doesn't do the trick it will be repeated 2 or 3 times a week from now on. You know I'll have no problem finding people to spank you and if I have the time that won't even be necessary."

My mouth dropped open. "But Mistress it will hurt so much." "Good" was her reply. Master Terry should be there to spank you anytime now." With that she hung up. I was stunned. 10 good spankings in one day may be some kind of personal record. I tried to think back to the most spankings I've had in a day and if it was a day that included one of those sex parties, I'd say 15 but the spankings I often got at a sex party was short and often not that forceful. Oh my gosh. Suddenly I wasn't horny at all but concerned, then I heard the doorbell, oh oh, here comes another spanking.

I got out of bed, naked of course and put my slippers on. I hurried to the door. Looking through the peephole I saw Master Terry. I let him in, keeping my eyes down of course. "Your owner asked me to come by and give you a good spanking. I hear you were forgetful again." "Yes sir" I muttered, still stunned by my Mistress' news. "Very well, go fetch my favorite paddle, the brown and gold one." "Yes Sir."

The brown and gold paddle was a gift to my mistress from her mother who was also a mistress. It's about 2 feet long and maybe a third of an inch thick. It has holes in it and a black leather handle. It's nasty but I have a very tough butt.

I got back to the living room and Master Terry had already gotten out of his cloths. "Crawl to me slave". I quickly got down on all 4s and crawled to him, giving him the paddle. "Kneel in front of me slave, hands on my legs." I gave him the paddle. My mouth was now only a couple of feet from his cock. Unexpectedly I felt a tremendous urge to suck on it. My horniness had returned. "Suck" he ordered. Master Terry was pretty predictable. I would suck on his cock for a while as he spanked me with the long paddle. Fortunately I am well trained and won't clamp my teeth down on his manhood as he spanked. The intensity of his spanking at the moment was not that bad. He was after all being sucked and didn't want to tempt fate. I do have teeth. I knew from experience that he would soon stop spanking and play with my breasts as I sucked, invariably ordering me to cum. Oh god I can't wait. I lost track of how many spanks I was getting. I was however ready to cum but knew better than to try to ask. "Faster slave". My head bobbed up and down faster on his cock as I feverishly played with his balls. Mistress had always taught me to play with a man's balls while I was sucking on his cock. Holding a cane, she would watch me as I sucked on a cock to see if I would dare disobeyed her in that regard. (As I noted earlier, she is very strict.) If she thought I was not playing hard enough with a man's balls she would say "head up" and I would lift my head off of his cock and she would cane my bottom to everyone's delight.

Then it happened, Master Terry reached down and commenced playing with my d-cup breasts. He was always good at it and I could wait no longer. I stopped sucking momentarily and begged "please sir may I cum?" He said yes and I nearly saw stars. I had to keep sucking hard though or he'd stop playing with my breasts and immediately start my beating. I shuttered some and hesitated momentarily but caught myself and kept sucking as hard as I could. I thought I did quite an impressive job to be honest. I made gurgling noise as I sucked and came. My tits kept being played with, it was great. After about 5 minutes of heaven I was ordered over his lap as he sat on the couch. Oh that's right, the spanking, that's mainly what he's here for. Well at least I was recharged after that orgasm. Besides my butt was already broken in for the day, how bad could it be?

The other thing I wanted to mention is that Master Terry was a very sensual master and liked his sub/slave playmates to cum a lot. He is also a gentleman so he started the paddling easy and worked his way up to the hard stuff. "I hear you are being forgetful again and your owner wants to nip this in the bud." He was spanking now as he spoke. "Yes sir" I managed to say. He was spanking faster and harder now. BAM, BAM, SMACK, slap, slap, smoosh, slap, bam, BAM. He was spanking harder than usual and man it hurt. "I had a slave that was forgetful and this is just what I gave her. You cannot spank a forgetful slave too much." BAM, SMACK, SMACK, BAM, slap BAM, SMACK, SMACK. "Yes sir" I was now holding back tears and biting on a couch pillow. "ow, oh, pleassse no morre, oow, oh, ow" I mumbled. He then spoke "Your mistress insisted on me spanking you good and hard and that young lady is what I'm going to do." He was now spanking real hard and in rapid machine gun like fashion. That was it. The dam broke and I started softly crying. "I won't forrrggett sir I prooomise." I started kicking my legs a little but I knew better than to move my butt away. Darnn master Terry was strong too. Suddenly he stopped. I couldn't believe it. "Give me you right hand". I gave it to him and he pulled it across the small of my back, now he had made me more immobile. "Beg for the spanking to continue." "Please sir, spank me more." Like that was an easy thing for me to say. "You can do better than that" he roared. "Oh please sir paddle my ass until I have learned my lesson and will be a very good girl." Well I got my wish I guess and the paddling continued. SMACK, BAM, slap, BAM, SMACK, SMACK. "Owwee" was that me that just said that. Wow it was. "Legs spread" he ordered and I quickly spread my legs. He spanked in the areas down by the pussy, the areas that were still white, areas that Mistress hadn't even gotten too in her haste. Oh gosh, I have another spanking from Mistress coming up at lunchtime, and this one isn't even over yet. SMACK, BAM, slap, slap, BAM, SMACK, SMACK, slap. My ass cheeks were bouncing back and forth. Then suddenly he ordered me to cum. I went from "please stop, ow, ow, oh" to making guttural sounds and not feeling the paddle at all. "I'm cummingggg" I screamed as I rubbed his legs with my pussy as hard as I could, still the spanking went on, slap, BAM, SMACK, SMACK, SMACK, SMACK. He was spanking very evenly from one cheek to the next, upper cheek then lower cheek and some on the upper legs but I continued to cum as ordered; then suddenly the spanking stopped. His hand went down to my pussy and finger fucked me. I arched my back and came even harder for him. I don't know where he found all that energy but his fingers were going in and out of me like a dynamo. Finally he stopped. He then ordered me off his lap to continue sucking on his cock. I hesitated at first as my orgasm was still going on even though nothing was touching my pussy or clit. I worked my way to his cock. "Suck" he ordered and my mouth went back to work.

I rubbed my ass cheeks with one hand and played with his balls with the other. They once again my cheeks were hot and red. I was dying to look at them but knew better than to stop sucking. I was tasting a lot of Master Terry's ozze and knew what was coming soon. He came with a shout and filled my mouth with his cum. He held my head in place on his cock. "Faster slave" he ordered and forced my head deeper onto his cock. I drank down all his cum. For many minutes I knelt there making sure to drink down all off Master Terry's cum. Finally he got up, got dressed as we talked. "I hear you're getting 10 spankings today and that could be repeated soon". "Yes sir." "Well maybe I'll stop by again this week to give you another one." "Yes sir." Like I had a choice.

With his clothes back on Master Terry left and I went to the tall bathroom mirror to look at my pink butt. It still stung some but I came so hard during the spanking that I'd have to consider that spanking a breeze. I wish mistress would let me cum more often when she spanked me but my Mistress is strict, demanding and controlling. But she also pays the bills. Most of the orgasms I got from Mistress were when she was taking me with one of her strap-ons, something she enjoyed doing very much. She would start by taking me in my pussy, which I was required to exercise to keep nice and tight for her, and then take me in my ass. Mostly she took me in my ass but I came just as hard from being taken in either my pussy or ass.

Often the two of us would lay together naked in mistress' bed. Mistress is very proud of her property. Her hands would wander when laying in bed with her slave girl. Sometimes her fingertips caressed, other times her nails scraped as she explored her slave's body. My nipples would get a lot of attention. When mistress tired of such torment, perhaps she'd tie my hands together. She would then take her time choosing what toys to use on me next. Perhaps earlier I didn't move fast enough or I made too much noise, waking her from her nap. Or maybe she's just in the mood to paddle my butt. My ass is her property to do what she wishes with after all. She would bend me over her knee, flip up my short skirt, if I've been allowed to wear any clothes, and run her nails over my already well-spanked ass. Her spanking starts slow and gained momentum: slap, slap, slap, SMACK, SMACK, SMACK. Once my ass is a lovely shade of red she'll send me to fetch her crop, floggers and handcuffs. My bound hands are hooked to the ceiling high above my head, so I have to stretch up on my tiptoes. Then she works my body over with her crop and floggers, gentle taps punctuated with hard smacks. When she's done beating me, she lets me down. With my bound hands in front of me I am lead to her bed. She strips and lays down with her pussy on the edge of the bed. I am then ordered to pleasure her. She enjoys watching me wiggle into a position that allows me to put my tongue to good use.

With my well-spanked naked ass now sticking up and out, if someone else walks by I will inevitably get taken. Mistress likes to watch other mistress' use the strap-on on me and will invite them over to watch them do just that, often while I am sucking on her pussy. The problem can be that if he or she pounds me too hard from behind while taking me, I often can't keep my mouth on mistress' pussy adequately while eating her. It's not my fault but I will be the one getting punished.

Anyway, so there I was being all dreamy. I had to write some emails so I got on the computer and wrote away. Mistress' lunch break started at noon and it took her 15 minutes to drive over here and another 15 minutes to drive back. I had to have lunch ready soon. She would spank me first then eat. That way she had cooled off a bit before heading back to work as spanking me can make her work up a sweat. It was always the same. She would sit on the couch where master Terry spanked me, and then proceed to redden my butt there. It was 11:30 so I got all the implements she might want and put them on the coffee table in front of where she would spank me OTK. As she'll be in a hurry, it's doubtful she'll tie my hands together, even though she loves doing that before spanking me. As noon approached I made a plate of food for her, had something to eat myself and went and knelt by the couch in anticipation of my spanking.

I was only there for about 2 minutes when she walked in and immediately sat in front of me on the couch. "Over my lap young lady" she ordered and I crawled over her lap as I had done so many times before. "Your ass is still warm, nice, but it's not particularly red. Let's see if we can change that." Oh I knew she could. "Now which of these shall I use." Mistress first picked up a black leather slapper but put it down instead opting for a ping pong paddle. She rubbed my butt tenderly with her hands for a bit, then with the paddle. "I see that between my spanking earlier and master Terry's spanking we're leaving our mark on your lovely ass. Perhaps after this day and night is done, you will have learned your lesson." "Yes maam."

Well the rubbing was fun while it lasted but then mistress started spanking in earnest. SMACK... BAM, slap, slap...BAM, SMACK...SMACK, BAM...BAM, slap, slap, slap. I started squirming. "Hold still slave or you'll spend the next 3 days in the cage except to work, serve and be punished." Gee, that didn't sound like fun. I quickly gained my composure and largely stayed put. SMACK, SMACK..BAM, BAM, slap, slap, BAM, SMACK, SMACK, SMACK, SMACK… BAM, slap. My butt by now was tender enough for me to really feel the swats. "Ow, ow, no please, ow, aw, aw, stop please, oh." "Music to my ears my dear" Mistress said as she started spanking me harder. "Oh please no, ow." I grabbed once again on to the couch cushion and held onto it with all my might. Fortunately my butt began acclimating to the blows and the pain tapered off some. Then mistress started with the irregular blows. I hate those. She'd rub my butt with the paddle then quickly raise it and bring it down on me, many times in rapid succession. "Now let's see how fast I can give you 50". I didn't just hear 50 did I? SMACK, SMACK, BAM, slap, BAM, slap, slap, BAM, SMACK. I was squirming as the blows really hurt. I tried to stay in place as much as possible. I raised and lowered my butt some from the pain. RAT, TAT, TAT, BAM, BAM, SMACK, BAM. "Stop pleasssssse Mistress, I'll be gooooodd." 29, 30, 31, 32, she counted out. I started kicking my feet some but caught myself and held back as much as I could. I cried out as she started the 40s. She was now spanking with all her might. "Ow, no mistress, stop, oww, ow." Abruptly mistress pushed me off her lap and dropped the paddle. I rubbed my scorching bottom. "Kiss my foot." I crawled over to mistress and kissed her left shoe. "Lick it slave". I lathered it up with my tongue, then she pulled her foot away and bent over to inspect her work as I held my naked ass up in the air. "Not bad for a quickie. Tonight your tits get it also and it will be an all night affair. I'll give you all the spankings left to make 10 for the day." Mistress went into the kitchen to eat. I stayed there on my hands and knees. Soon she came out and grabbed her car keys. "You're going to have more visitors this afternoon. You'll take their punishment and serve them." "Who will be punishing me maam?" "Mistress Tammy and Master Brian. I may find someone else to punish you also. Mistress Tammy should be here anytime. I need to go. Now go stand in the corner and wait for Mistress Tammy." "Yes Maam." I stopped rubbing my butt and walked over to the corner putting my nose against where both walls meet. I heard the front door close as Mistress left.

My butt was sore, three good spankings in this short of a period was the real thing. I wanted to go look in the tall bathroom mirror at how red my butt was but my orders were to stay in the corner until Mistress Tammy got there.

Mistress Tammy was a good friend of my Mistress and they have shared slaves before. I knew what a visit from Mistress Tammy meant, a tit whipping. Mistress Tammy loved to play with and beat tits. I've never seen anyone quite like her when it comes to that. She has a tit fetish I think. On the other hand she sure knows how to make them feel good. I hope that today will be one of those times.

Chapter Three

Sure enough I didn't have to wait long. Mistress had left the door unlock and soon Mistress Tammy walked in. "Hello my dear, your mistress requested my assistance in punishing you and I was oh so eager to be of service. Aren't you grateful?" "Yes maam" What was I going to say. I haven't whipped those lovely tits of yours in a while have I?" "No maam." "Frankly I've missed them." I see you're undressed, good."

Mistress Tammy was herself quite good looking. She was a professional femdom that made a living from it. When it came to sex though she much preferred girls to guys. "Come kneel in front of me my dear." I took my nose away from the corner and walked over to her. She was sitting on the couch where I had recently gotten spanked. "Kneel". I knelt in front of her and close to her with my hands behind my head. She caressed and played with my tits. She had always really liked them. "Up higher on your knees young lady" she ordered. My breasts were now at her mouth level and she began sucking away on them. I begged to cum but she ignored me, as if she never even heard it. She pulled both nipples into her mouth and sucked on them. My knees buckled from the pleasure. I don't think it was an orgasm but I continued begging for permission to cum, no such luck. Unfortunately she was a Mistress that was also into orgasm denial, unless she was taking me with the strap-on, which she was almost sure to do later on. I could already tell that she was horny but at least it meant I would spend some time eating her first, thus at least putting off the inevitable tit torture.

Mistress Tammy then released my tits and pulled me towards her by the back of my head to kiss her. She had done this before but I had forgotten about it. She stood up and removed her clothing. She then leaned back on the couch, spread her legs and ordered me to pleasure her.

I had been taught that when I am eating someone or sucking a cock, I am to stick my butt up and out so it can be enjoyed and otherwise used by others. By using long implements my ass can be beaten by the person I'm pleasuring. I hadn't seen it when I had originally come over but next to her, Mistress Tammy had put her long red flogger. I found Mistress' clit and sucked on it. I felt her shutter and heard the moans. I really could eat pussy well. Everybody knew that. "Harder slave" I heard her say as she rested the flogger on my back. I lapped down mistress' pussy juice, spreading her pussy lips as I licked and sucked. This mistress really took care of herself. She ate well, worked out, didn't smoke, etc and I could tell by how good her pussy juice tasted. I love good tasting pussy juice and I lapped it up eagerly. I felt her cumming, then, suddenly she began flogging my upturned butt as she moaned in ecstasy. FLOP, FLACK...SMACK, CRACK...CRACK, BAM...FLOP, SMACK. The flogger kept landing mostly on my butt but also she flogged my back. She wasn't beating me particularly hard, besides I didn't care cause I loved sucking down her tasty pussy juice and the beating was just getting me hornier.

Suddenly it stopped. "head up young lady." I forced myself to stop eating her and took my head away from her wonderful pussy. I kept my eyes on it hoping that being away from it would be just a temporary thing but it was not to be. "Your Mistress tells me your forgetfulness has returned and she wants it to end.' "Yes Maam." "Clearly then you need quite a bit of discipline for such a thing. We're going to start with a spanking and then a tit whipping. You know how I love to whip those gorgeous tits of yours." "Yes mistress." "Give me your hands." I clapped my hands together in front of her lap and she tied them securely together. She motioned me to lay over her lap which I did. She began rubbing my already tender butt. "Legs spread". I spread my legs about 2 feet wide. She then stuck her finger up my pussy. Wow did it ever easily slide in. "Wow, you are one wet slavegirl. Very good. But no you're not cumming yet." Too bad but that's the way these mistresses are, so much orgasm denial.

Mistress started my spanking with her hand. She went right to work too, SMACK, SMACK, BAM, BAM, slap, slap, BAM, SMACK, SMACK, SMACK, SMACK, SMACK, BAM, slap. I lost count as to how many spanks. I had also forgotten how much Mistress Tammy liked to spank with her hand. Now she was spanking hard, smiling down on me as I squirmed and moaned. "I don't accept forgetfulness in a slave so why should your owner? "I understand maam" was all I could muster. BAM, BAM, CRACK, CRACK, slap, slap, BAM, SMACK, SMACK. My ass was tender from the day's abuse so I was feeling this more than usual. I kicked my legs a bit. Mistress was really laying it on fast and furious. Then suddenly I found myself on the verge of cumming. I knew Mistress wouldn't let me cum so why ask. I continued to yelp, moan and squirm. Now I thought I might cry then suddenly I started cumming even though I didn't mean to. I tried hard not to move my pelvis in a manner that would give away that I was cumming without permission but suddenly mistress' scolding and spanks meant a lot less. Then mistress Tammy stopped using her hand, reached for a strap and continued the deluge on my ass, rubbing it periodically to admire her work. I had a nice controlled orgasm as she scolded and spanked me. SMACK, BAM...BAM, slap, slap, BAM, SMACK..SMACK, SMACK, slap. I turned back to look at my ass and it was red. "Eyes forward" mistress scowled giving me 5 really hard strokes to punctuate it. The spanking now was really hurting and as I had lost concentration, I also lost my orgasm, now all I felt was pain. "Ow, noo mistress, stop, oow, ow." I pounded the couch in pain. Mistress had never spanked me so hard. "Hold your ass still slave." I hadn't realized it but I had lifted my butt up some to avoid the spanks. Wow, that was a bad idea. Mistress went back to work on my ass and upper legs, this time with a medium size rubber paddle. "Ow, ooh, ooh, pleassee maam, I'llll be good." Dozens of spanks later I was crying. I can take a really hard spanking but all this attention to my posterior was really getting to me. Then suddenly it stopped.

"Kneel" was the order and I eagerly knelt in front of her as I rubbed my butt cheeks. "I see we have some tears here" mistress said looking into my eyes. "Good. I believe the message is getting through to you." "Yes maam" I moaned while rubbing my naked, sore bottom. "Now it's time to give those lovely tits of yours the same kind of attention." Oh great, but at least my butt would get a rest for a change.

I had been trained to easily cum from breast stimulation. I am so proud of my breasts. They give me and others so much pleasure. They can take quite a beating too. Mistress Tammy specialized in tit torture so I suspect my tits would be red soon.

As I knelt in front of her, Mistress Tammy untied my wrists and ordered me to turn around and put my wrists behind my back. She tied my hands behind my back and then ordered me to face her again. She then tied my boobs fairly tightly together at their base. My tits were even firmer than usual now. Their nipples quickly hardened. Mistress pinched both nipples hard waking me from my dreamy state and making me yelp. "What is my favorite color for your tits slave?" "Red maam." "You're darn right, especially if you're being punished. What do your tits exist for?" "To be played with and beaten maam." "Good girl."

Mistress then took out a short tit flogger and proceeded to lightly whip my tits with it as I continued to kneel in front of her. I closed my eyes instinctively but the flogger never came anywhere close to my face. Mistress Tammy really knew how to whip tits. Mistress started to swing from a further distance away thus increasing the velocity. I could tell this was something she really enjoyed doing. She started playing with one of her nipples as she was whipping the other one. This flogging went on for about 5 minutes. Mistress then put the flogger down and took up the same slapper she had earlier used on my butt. She pulled my head back by the hair exposing my breasts more and proceeded to spank them for real.

Slap, slap, slap, slap, slap, SMACK, SMACK, BAM, slap, slap. Mistress concentrated spanking the fleshing mounds of the left breast, reaching out, grabbing it by the nipple and separating it from the right breast so more off my large breast was free to spank. It did sting but also felt sinfully good. "A forgetful slave girl needs to be a well beaten slavegirl. Isn't that right young lady?" "Yess maaam." I managed to say. Smack...slap, slap, slap, SMACK, SMACK, BAM, slap. Mistress pinched my left nipple as she held it making me wince but then she twisted it in-between her fingers giving me pleasure. She probably didn't even realize she was playing with the nipple in such a pleasurable way. Giving breasts pleasure and pain is just her nature. I sure wasn't going to complain. Then she let go of my left nipple and got a hold of the right nipple, pulling the right breast out to the right, separating it from its twin, allowing more of it to be beaten. Slap, slap, slap, SMACK, SMACK, BAM, slap. "Do you know how much I enjoy beating your tits young lady?" "Ow, oh...a lot maam." "Girl do I ever." Slap, slap, slap, SMACK, SMACK, BAM, slap, slap. Blow after blow continued to rain down on my breasts, making them pink and tender. Mistress pulled up my right breast by the nipple and concentrated her beating on the underside. It did hurt but frankly I got more pleasure from a tit whipping from her than when she spanks my ass. I glanced down at my breasts and they were getting red. Suddenly I blurted it out "Mistress please may I cum?". The whipping stopped suddenly as mistress looked at me somewhat puzzled. "Wow, you are an amazing slave and I love how masochistic you are." Then she got very serious and got close to me and bellowed "but you know slave that you may not cum. You are being punished and you should know better than to even hope for it." She them grabbed both of my large nipples together with one hand and pulled my breasts up exposing their soft underbelly, going to work on them both at once with the slapper and spanking them hard now. "Ow, ohh no mistress, ow, oww, oh pleeaaseee mistress." Slap...slap, slap...slap, slap, SMACK, BAM...slap, slap. She let go of my tits and they flopped down in front of her. She then proceeded to spank their upper front. "You know how much I love whipping your tits" "Oh yes mistress, ow, ow, oh, ow." This was really hurting now and I wasn't going to be allowed to cum so I was going to just have to take it.

My breasts were now a shade of red and Mistress Tammy stopped. I thought my tit whipping was over but I was wrong. "Turn around slave." I turned around obediently and knelt there as she untied my wrists. Then in my stupor I remembered that there was another position for me and my tits to be whipped in...and more.

Mistress, herself now naked, lead me over to the half table. I was ordered to lay on my back on it. It was a familiar position for me. My pussy and ass were on the table's edge and thus would be easy to play with and take. My back and head were laying on the table. Mistress tied each leg to the table's built-in stirrups. The ankles and thighs got tied to the stirrups. A strap came over my lower pelvis to keep it in place and straps held each arm in place. I was now quite vulnerable and immobile.

My mistress put me here often and left me here for her and other's pleasure. My legs are positioned such that I can be easily spanked and taken both in my pussy and ass. I was also blindfolded. But for the time being Mistress Tammy was a lot more interested in finishing the job she started with my breasts. Now though she would use the big black flogger to beat them. This part would make me cry and leave my pussy dripping.

Mistress bend down to my pussy and sucked the copious amount of cum out of it. "You know what's coming now young lady don't you." "Yes maam" I think I said. She raised the flogger and CRACK. "Ow". CRACK, CRACK..SMACK. This is a big room so mistress could raise up the big flogger and let it fly. CRACK, CRACK..SMACK, BAM...SMACK, BAM. I was now whimpering and trying to move away but to no avail. I was held too tightly in place and could go nowhere. BAM, SMACK, BAM. Mistress was working up a sweat and loving every second of it. "Are you still going to be a forgetful slave?" "No Misstresss". I was so exposed and I knew by now my pussy was dripping wet. I couldn't wait for her to take me with her strap-on like she always did. And she would take me for a long time too. I held onto that thought as the blows rained down on my chest. "Mistress, please, oww, oww, ahhh." Mistress was very skilled and the flogger never landed more than a couple of inches above my breasts. Finally it was over but I kept whimpering.

She now played with my sensitive breasts with her gloved hands grabbing, kneading, twisting, turning and holding them. "I am so proud of my work. Your breasts are so much fun to work with. You know your tits are my favorite tits to whip." Oh lucky me. "Thank you maam." I whimpered. Mistress bent down and lightly bite my nipples one by one, also sucking on them and playing with my breasts more. She was so proud of her work and loved my tits. Suddenly I remembered what was to come next, yes, it could be the highlight of my day.

I looked down at my chest and it was a light shade of red. My nipples were hot and sensitive. I heard mistress doing something and I looked over at her. She had put on one of her strap-ons and was coming over to my exposed holes. First she got out some Vaseline and used her finger to lubricate my anus. She inserted her finger deep into it making me moan in anticipation. She then cleaned off her finger with a paper towel. "Beg for it slave" she ordered. "Mistress please take me with your big black strap-on". "You can do better than that." "Mistress I'm begging, please take me with your big black strap-on and fuck me hard because I've been such a bad slave. I need to be fucked hard by Mistress to clear my head and not be forgetful." Then she entered my pussy. Immediately I began begging to cum, which she allowed me to do.

Mistress grabbed my upper legs to hold me in place while she pounded my pussy with her strap-on. I came so hard. I lost track of what time it was. "Come harder slut" she roared and I did just that pumping my hips against her as she took me. I couldn't wait for her to take me in my ass even though it was a fairly thick strap-on. "You like how this feels in that naughty little cunt of yours don't you slave." "Yes maam" I stammered. She pounded me harder and buried the strap-on in my pussy, just leaving it there for a few moments as she gyrated her hips, making it move from side to side. I was so wet that it slide easily in my pussy. "Wow, you're one soaking wet little slave girl." I couldn't answer though I think I tried. I was cumming so hard. A few minutes after she started taking me, she was cumming too. About then she pulled out of my pussy and stuck the strap-on in my ass. "Ohhhhh mistress, yes, thank you….ohhh." She started taking me slowly in the ass at first but built up speed and after a couple of minutes was pounding my butthole with vigor. I felt no pain, just waves of ecstasy.

Mistress finished taking me a while later, cleaned off her equipment as I lay tied down exhausted and helpless. She left me there with my spread legs up in the air. My tits a light shade of red and my ass sore and tender. "I hope you will learn your lesson today young lady but then again I hope you don't as I do love these sessions so much. Your owner said to leave you like this as master Brian will be here soon to do as she wishes with you. What have you to say?" "Thank you maam for disciplining and taking me." "Good girl." With that she left.

Chapter Four

There I was alone and tied down waiting for the next person to punish and ravage me. It wasn't that big of a deal as I've been on this table like this often. I sure hope I don't have to go to the bathroom while no one is here though. Fortunately it's usually not a problem. Mistress always talked about putting a mirror on the wall across from my upturn legs, ass and pussy. That would be nice as I could see how red my ass was getting. Strapped down like this I could only move myself some from the tits up as my arms were strapped down which limited my movement. My blindfold was still on me.

Master Brian really liked to fuck me in the ass. I don't think he had ever taken me in my pussy. A drawback to Doms in regard to the position I was in strapped down to this table, is that it is difficult for me to suck on their cocks. Mistresses can get on the table and sit on my face for me to pleasure them. Master Brian has had me in this position before so I was expecting the usual ass whipping and ass fucking. I didn't really like Master Brain that much and I don't think he's a particularly good lover but I had no say in the matter.

Then I heard someone enter, man I hope that's Master Brian, and I could tell from his voice that it was. "Wow, look at you. All ready to be beaten and taken." I wasn't sure if I was suppose to answer so I didn't say anything. I heard him undressing. "I'm going to fuck you silly bitch. I heard about your forgetfulness, well I'm here to beat it out of you." I heard noises like he was getting something together to spank me with. "Any requests for what I should spank you with?" "Your hand sir?" "Nice try but you know how I like the belt." No not the belt. He had a wide leather belt that he had had for ages. The rustling I heard must have been him taking that it off his pants. He likes to wear it around when he's going to whip a slave with it. He looked over and felt my ass. "How many spankings have you gotten today young lady?" "Four so far sir." "Wow, your ass looks surprisingly good for all that, you always could take quite a spanking." "Thank you sir." He then came over and began playing with my tits, each hand on a tit. "Man I love these tits, especially when they have such a nice red hue like now. What do you say slave?" "Thank you sir." Getting my tits played with again felt good. They were still tender from the tit whipping though but gratefully were gifting me with lots of pleasure. I started to groan seductively and move my head slowly back and forth. I knew he wouldn't let me cum so I didn't even try asking.

"Guess what I'm going to beat your ass with?" "Your belt sir?" "Good girl, you remember well." I heard some rustling then I felt him lubing up my anus for after the beating. Then suddenly I felt nothing. That's trouble. Past my upturn legs and exposed pussy I heard him whipping the air with the belt. Oh man, this is not good. Then he lightly swung the belt against my ass. It was just the start of things to come. It would be my worst beating of the day. SMACK, BAM, BAM…SMACK, SMACK, SMACK, BAM. I yelled out from the beginning, making his cock hard no doubt. He grabbed my legs and drew himself closer to me. The whipping continued. SMACK, SMACK, SMACK, BAM, BAM, BAM, BAM. I tried to move my ass but it was too securely in place. Then I realized I was crying "Ow, ow, no please, ow, aw, aw, stop please, ohhh, nnnno." He pulled my ass out as far as the pelvic strap would allow all in an effort to expose as much ass as possible. SMACK, SMACK, SMACK, BAM, BAM. Master Brian was in heaven, he is a sadistic Dom with cart blanche to punish a wayward slavegirl. I could not escape the blows that were raining down on my ass. "I'mmm begging masterr, pleaseee. BAM, SLAP, Slap, BAM…SMACK. Tears were running down my cheeks. I can usually take a good beating but as sensitive as my ass was from the days' previous onslaught and this brute of a master wailing away on my tender ass with a big belt, was too much. I don't think my mistress would even be happy about this. I know this would leave marks on my ass."Masterrrr, pleaaaasse, oh, aw, pleassse stoppp pleaaaase, oh."

Something on my ass felt different then I realized that the beating had stopped. Master Brian had also whipped my upper legs, something mistress will not like. Leaving marks on my legs, or on anyone else's property, is not good etiquette. I continued to cry. I didn't hear back from him but I heard him making himself harder and I knew the beating was over. He would concentrate now on my asshole. I felt him come up to me, grab both my hips and thrust himself into me….."ohhhh" I shuttered glad to be feeling another type of sensation but my ass was still on fire.

Master Brian always grunted a lot when he fucked. It sounded real animal but a cock in my ass was a welcome change and soon I felt an orgasm coming on. Oh god, I hope this meany will let me cum. "Permission to cum sir please." No answer. "Please sir may I cum….oh please, please." I hate him. I tried hard to not cum and I was able to stifle the orgasm. Doms like him give BDSM a bad name as far as I was concerned. I don't get taken by him often and was going to talk to mistress about him, still his cock pounding my ass did feel real good, even if I couldn't cum. I laid back and enjoyed it. At least 5 of my beatings for the day were over-with.

See volume 2 for slave sarah's next 5 spankings of the day.

www.ingramcontent.com/pod-product-compliance
Lightning Source LLC
Chambersburg PA
CBHW070611290526
45790CB00002B/869